A Practical Guide to Forensic Mental Health Consultation through Aphorisms and Caveats

A Practical Guide to Forensic Mental Health Consultation through Aphorisms and Caveats

Daniel P. Greenfield, MD, MPH, MS, FASAM

Seton Hall University

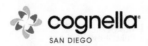

cognella®
SAN DIEGO

Bassim Hamadeh, CEO and Publisher

Amy Smith, Senior Project Editor

Jeanine Rees, Production Editor

Jess Estrella, Senior Graphic Designer

Kylie Bartolome, Licensing Associate

Natalie Piccotti, Director of Marketing

Kassie Graves, Senior Vice President of Editorial

Jamie Giganti, Director of Academic Publishing

Cover image Copyright © 2021 iStockphoto LP/Nastco.
Cover image Copyright © 2011 Depositphotos/Morphart.
Cover image Copyright © 2012 Depositphotos/lhfgraphics.

Printed in the United States of America.

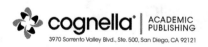

3970 Sorrento Valley Blvd., Ste. 500, San Diego, CA 92121

As with my previous volumes, this book is dedicated to my family, children, and grandchildren, who I hope will be amused and informed by it.

I also dedicate this book to the colleagues, students, trainees, and friends who shared their interests and experiences with me over the years and gave me the basis for this book.

Lawyers, I suppose, were children once.
—Charles Lamb (1775–1834)

Contents

THIS BOOK IS a "must read" for anyone seeking to prepare a written report and/or testify in court as an expert witness.

I served for 25 years as a judge in the Superior Court of New Jersey—15 years presiding over jury trials in the Criminal Division, 5 years presiding over non-jury trials in the Family Division, and 5 years presiding over non-jury civil trials in the Chancery Division. In a significant percentage of the over 600 trials I was involved in, expert witnesses prepared reports and testified before me. Many of the expert witnesses who appeared before me were forensic mental health professionals (FMHPs), including the author of this book, Daniel P. Greenfield, MD, MPH, MS, FASAM, and Clinical Professor of Neuroscience (Psychiatry) at Seton Hall University (South Orange, New Jersey). I have known Dr. Greenfield since we went to high school together, although he has to respect me because I was one grade ahead of him.

This book is a succinct but comprehensive step-by-step practical guide for FMHPs. It is well-organized, and it is written with humility, humanity, and humor, and without a trace of hubris. The book uses aphorisms (pithy observations that contain general truths, such as "If it ain't broke, don't fix it"). And the book also uses caveats (warnings or provisos of specific stipulations, conditions, or limitations, such as "*Caveat emptor*" [Let the buyer beware]). Through the use of these aphorisms and caveats, Dr. Greenfield covers all the bases as to what makes an expert witness effective.

Those bases, in my humble opinion, are as follows:

1. Qualification: The expert must be qualified and knowledgeable in his or her field by virtue of both training and experience.

2. Communication: The expert must be able to communicate to the trier of facts (the jury or the judge) in terms that the non-expert can understand, without using unnecessary technical jargon on the one hand, and talking down to laypersons as if they were second graders on the other hand.

3. Objectivity: The expert must be objective and reasonable when explaining the facts on which the opinions they espouse are based. The expert must never be a "hired gun."

4. Credibility: If the expert is qualified, able to communicate effectively, and objective, they will be best able to be credible or believable to the triers of facts.

Since he covered all the bases, I would say Dr. Greenfield hit a home run with this book.

Here are just a few examples of what I call "little nuggets" Dr. Greenfield uses in this book to get some of these concepts across:

- "As in therapy, sex, and life in general, preparation is everything."
- In the interview or examination conducted by the forensic mental health professional, what is most essential is "privacy, quiet, non-interference from others, and an environment in which information and ideas can be freely exchanged."
- "I am an advocate for my expert opinion in this matter, not for either side."
- When testifying on cross-examination, "Don't argue with the cross-examiner, but hold your position, when reasonable, and be assertive without being aggressive."

As I said at the outset: Read this book!

—*The Honorable R. Benjamin Cohen, JD, JSC (Retired)*
Superior Court of New Jersey (Essex Vicinage)
February 2021

PREFACE

*While Wile E. Coyote is by no stretch of the imagination
a superhero, I have to admit that it was this hapless
villain ... who first got me thinking about ... physics. ...*
—L. Krauss, from the Foreword of *The Physics
of Superheroes* (see Selected References)

THE INSPIRATION FOR this book comes from *The Physics of Superheroes* (2006), a straightforward undergraduate textbook of physics, authored by James Kakalios, PhD, at the time Professor of Physics and Astronomy at the University of Minnesota. This introductory textbook is based on comic book and graphic novel characters, and illustrates, for example,

- how Plastic Man embodies elasticity theory and Young's modulus,

- how Iceman's and Storm's powers explain thermodynamics, and

- how Superman's powers illustrate classical Newtonian mechanics.

Some time ago, I was re-reading *The Physics of Superheroes* and I realized that much of what I know and do as a forensic psychiatrist comes from nontechnical and practical sources: from experiences "in the trenches," from listening to and speaking with colleagues and evaluees, from mentors, and from paying attention to aphorisms and caveats encountered and overheard in the field.

Out of that realization came the topic for a panel presentation at the American College of Forensic Psychology's 35th Annual Symposium in 2018. During the brainstorming for that panel, two colleagues and I almost simultaneously agreed that a concise, practical, and minimally technical "how-to" guide to forensic mental health consultation practice, based on and structured by aphorisms and caveats in the forensic mental health consultation practice world, could be a useful contribution to the field.

In due course, we created the panel presentation based on aphorisms and caveats. We structured the presentation to follow the flow of the forensic mental health consultation process, which we divided into several categories and stages, as follows:

- Engagement
- Preparation
- The Interview
- Collecting Your Thoughts
- The Report
- Testifying PRN
- On Cross-Examination
- Collecting Your Fees
- Wrapping Up

The presentation went well. Then, with the encouragement of Deborah Miller, Executive Director of the American College of Forensic Psychology, the presentation was been expanded into this book.

Distinguishing between *clinical/therapeutic* forensic mental health practice and *consulting* forensic mental health practice, this book is primarily focused on and intended for the latter.[1] The distinctions between these two types of practice include the following:

- *Clinical/therapeutic* forensic mental health practice involves clinical evaluation, treatment, and management of individuals in forensic populations such as correctional settings (jails, prisons, and penitentiaries). Such mental health professionals, however, must often serve as **forensic consultants** for their correctional patients at criminal, legal, and administrative events, such as hearings, parole and probation conferences and meetings, and the like.[2]

- *Consulting* forensic mental health practice, on the other hand, involves responding to clinical questions posed by counsel and/or the court relevant to legal concerns, such as (1) inferences about an individual's

---

1 To avoid confusion, I will refer to all types of individuals of all disciplines—psychiatrists, psychologists, social workers, licensed professional counselors (LPCs), physician assistants (PAs), advanced practice nurses (APNs), and others—involved in this work as "forensic mental health professionals" or "FMHPs" throughout this book.
2 Generally, this practice is inadvisable, although sometimes unavoidable. See Chapter 1.

underlying mental state and psychiatric/neuropsychiatric condition during various periods of time pertaining to such issues as criminal responsibility, competency to stand trial, and future dangerousness in criminal law; (2) psychiatric, psychological, and emotional responses to different types of exposures and experiences, such as accidents, alleged workplace misadventures, and medical treatment; pertaining to such issues as personal injury and employment law in civil law; and (3) psychiatric, psychological, and emotional concerns pertaining to divorce and custody issues in family law.

The nine chapters of this book are formatted to follow the flow of the consulting forensic mental health process. Each chapter corresponds to and describes a step in that process, and each chapter frames and discusses the step with an introductory table of aphorisms and caveats, followed by subsequent tables and text. Some of the tables apply to experts, some to counsel, and some to both. Commentary and discussion follow the aphorisms and caveats presented in the introductory table, expanding, explaining, and elaborating on the aphorisms and caveats themselves.

This book is offered to the forensic mental health community as a brief, useful, practical, minimally technical, occasionally humorous and facetious, lighthearted (hopefully), and non-scholarly *vade mecum* to help guide the neophyte as well as the experienced forensic expert through the shoals of forensic consultation. With this supplement to established and technical works such as Greenfield and Gottschalk's *Writing Forensic Reports: A Guide for Mental Health Professionals* (2008), Gutheil and Drogin's *The Mental Health Professional in Court: A Survival Guide* (2012), and Heilbrun's *Principles of Forensic Mental Health Assessment* (2001), the reader can avoid the most basic, first, and fundamental "caveat" which we cite, viz:

> *Lasciate ogni speranza, voi ch'entrata.*
> (Abandon all hope, ye who enter [the entrance to the Inferno].)
> —Dante's *Inferno* (1300)

Selected References

As a brief, minimally technical, and lighthearted piece, this volume is not intended to compete with, or replace, the many tomes, treatises, monographs, articles, journals, and the like having to do with evidence, expert testimony, and forensic mental health practice, with which the forensic literature is awash.

Rather, to the extent that given aphorisms and caveats in this book may be based on or reflect a documentable source of some sort, such sources, references, or citations will be noted in this Preface.

In that vein, selected references for the Preface appear below.

Brodsky, S. (2013). *Testifying in court: Guidelines and maxims for the expert witness* (2nd ed.). American Psychological Association.

Greenfield, D., & Gottschalk, J. (2008). *Writing forensic reports: A guide for mental health professionals*. Springer Publishing Company.

Gutheil, T., & Drogin, E. (2012). *The mental health professional in court: A survival guide*. American Psychiatric Publishing.

Heilbrun, K. (2001). *Principles of forensic mental health assessment*. Springer Publishing Company.

Kakalios, J. (2006). *The physics of superheroes*. Avery Publishing Group.

ACKNOWLEDGMENTS

T O THE EXTENT that forensic psychiatry as a legitimate academic, intellectual, and professional discipline has any credibility, the late Robert (Bob) L. Sadoff, MD—a pioneer in forensic psychiatry—was responsible. Bob was a friend and mentor to many of us, as well as a practitioner, senior academic, and trendsetter in forensic psychiatry for many years. I acknowledge his help and support over the years, and I miss him.

I also acknowledge the help and support of Edward J. Dougherty, EdD, MA, and Marc L. Zimmermann, MP, PhD. Ed, Marc, and I had the idea for and presented a panel on "Aphorisms and Caveats" at a national symposium of the American College of Forensic Psychology. That panel turned out to be the forerunner to this book.

To the Honorable R. Benjamin Cohen, JD, JSC (retired)—an old friend from many years ago in whose court I have testified as an expert witness and with whom I later reconnected as a friend—I am grateful for his Foreword to this book. Ben has a terrific sense of humor, which has served him well as a judge and attorney, and which is apparent from his Foreword.

I am particularly grateful to Joann Codella, my dedicated assistant and typist at the Department of Physician Assistant at Seton Hall University, who worked long, hard, and very well on the manuscript for this book, making it possible.

Thanks, too, to Joan Van der Veen, my private office manager, whose background and experience in publishing and graphics made her an invaluable asset with the production of this and previous books.

To Cognella Academic Publishing's Kassie Graves, Vice President, Editorial; Amy Smith, Senior Project Editor; and their staff, who made the process of working with them an efficient, careful, stimulating, rewarding, cooperative, educational, and even enjoyable experience: Thank you all very much.

Finally, I acknowledge the support and encouragement of my friends and colleagues at Seton Hall University. For reasons I do not understand, they pressed me for "war stories" about forensic practice and testimony, and told me that putting lessons learned from these stories into a book would be a good idea.

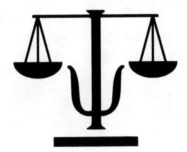

T HE GRAPHIC ON the cover of this book employs a symbol for forensic psychology/psychiatry. This particular symbol is widely used and recognized in forensic psychiatry, psychology, and other mental health sciences. It employs the Greek letter *psi* as the symbol of psychology/psychiatry combined with a depiction of a scale or balance as a metaphor for the law.

Psi is the next-to-last letter of the Greek alphabet. Psi represents the principles of human behavior, psychology and psychiatry ("psi," or "mind," or "psyche;" and "logos," or "study," also from the Greek).

The scales of justice, from the ancient Roman goddess of justice, Justitia, are a familiar graphic that represents the "weighing" of two sides of an argument and the equal, unbiased administration of the law.

In American- and English-based jurisprudence, the areas of the law to which forensic psychology/psychiatry may apply most frequently include the following:[1]

---

1 For an overview of these topics, the reader is referred to Chapters 1 and 2 (pages 3–16) of Greenfield, D. P., & Gottschalk, J. A. (2009). *Writing forensic reports: A guide for mental health professionals.* Springer Publishing Company.

IMG 0.1: Copyright © by ClipartMax.

- Criminal law: In the past, inferences about underlying mental states and psychological, psychiatric, and neuropsychiatric conditions during alleged criminal acts in terms of criminal responsibility and potential psychiatric defenses; at present, inferences about criminal competency; and in the future, inferences of future dangerousness

- Civil law: psychiatric, psychological, and neuropsychiatric effects, if applicable, of personal injury, workplace exposure and experiences, occupational exposures, and others, as well as professional liability and alleged malpractice)

- Family law: divorce, custody, and related issues

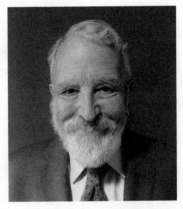

DANIEL P. GREENFIELD, MD, MPH, MS, FASAM is a practicing psychiatrist, addiction medicine specialist, and preventive medicine specialist. He was educated at Oberlin College, the University of North Carolina, the University of London, Cornell University Medical Center, Rutgers University, and Harvard University.

In addition to his clinical and forensic practice, Dr. Greenfield formerly taught at the Albert Einstein College of Medicine as an attending physician and at Montefiore Medical Center (Bronx, New York) as Clinical Associate Professor of Psychiatry and Behavioral Science.

Dr. Greenfield currently teaches at Seton Hall University, where he is Clinical Professor of Neuroscience (Psychiatry) at the JFK Neuroscience Institute Hackensack Meridian Health/JFK University Medical Center (South Orange, Nutley, and Edison, New Jersey).

Dr. Greenfield has lectured, published, and testified widely in areas of his background, training, and expertise in academic, business, community, courtroom, government, and professional forums, as well as on television and radio.

A Practical Guide to Forensic Mental Health Consultation through Aphorisms and Caveats is Dr. Greenfield's latest book. Other books by Dr. Greenfield include:

- *Prescription Drug Abuse and Dependence: How Prescription Drug Abuse Contributes to the Drug Abuse Epidemic* (1995)
- (with J. A. Gottschalk) *Writing Forensic Reports: A Guide for the Mental Health Professional* (2008)
- *A Primer of Psychiatry for NonPsychiatrists* (2021)
- *Psychopharmacology for NonPsychiatrists: A Primer* (2022; in press)

Dr. Greenfield can be reached at dpgreenfieldmdpsychiatry@msn.com.

AUTHOR'S DISCLAIMER

T HE FIELDS OF forensic mental health practice discussed, alluded to, and referenced in this book are dynamic fields, constantly changing and advancing, so that particular points, suggestions, aphorisms, and/or caveats made in this book may not apply in a particular case or cases. For these reasons, the reader is encouraged to supplement their knowledge by consulting applicable sources and references, including books, textbooks, articles, monographs, electronic databases, other Internet sources, and other such resources. A number of such sources are given in the Selected References in the Preface of this book, and sources are also cited in footnotes throughout the book.

Concerning discussion and commentary about the various aphorisms and caveats presented in this book, none of this information or commentary should be construed or taken as legal advice. Not being an attorney or legal professional, the author of this book is not competent to give such advice or opinions, which can only be given by a licensed attorney or qualified legal professional.

CHAPTER 1

Engagement

The Rules of the Game[1]

THE GAME IS afoot!"[2] Holmes and Watson—in *The Adventure of the Abbey Grange*—have just been contacted by Stanley Hopkins and are en route by train to the Abbey Grange in Marsham, Kent, to investigate the presumed death of Sir Eustace Brackenstall. Holmes had previously been retained by Hopkins "seven times, and on each occasion his summons has been entirely justified."[3] The "Great Detective" had a track record with Mr. Hopkins, which made the "engagement" phase of his consultation that much easier for all concerned.

Not all consulting forensic mental health professionals (FMHPs) have that advantage. Often enough, the FMHP has first been contacted, for example, by counsel's client—or in some other circuitous way—having "found you on Google and calling you on my own on behalf of the attorney because they are too busy to do it themselves. I hope you don't mind. Do you do that kind of work?"

Whether you mind or not, this method of contact puts the prospective FMHP off, and also puts them in the position of not knowing the potential consultee attorney or judge. The FMHP will need to establish a relationship with the potential consultee, and will need to deal with the myriad concerns, issues, and potential problems depicted in Table 1.2 (below), and—as a practical matter—in the rest of this book. So, the earliest of the aphorisms and caveats to be discussed in this book becomes obvious.

---

1 Page 636 in Doyle, A. C. (1930). *The complete Sherlock Holmes.* Doubleday & Company.
2 Of all 54 stories and 4 novels in the Sherlock Holmes canon of Sir Arthur Conan Doyle, the phrase "Watson, the game is afoot!" appears only once, despite its popularity with the reading public.
3 Ibid.

First things first: "aphorisms" and "caveats" are defined below, in Table 1.1.

TABLE 1.1   Definitions[4]

Aphorism—a pithy observation that contains a general truth. Example: "If it ain't broke, don't fix it."

Caveat—a warning or proviso of specific stipulations, conditions, or limitations. Example: *Caveat emptor* ("Let the buyer beware").

Next, in presenting the goals and objectives for the panel discussion on which this book is based, four points describe how careful the prospective FMHP must be in engaging in that process. The four points are the following:

1. "**Advise** about the parameters and pitfalls of taking on forensic mental health consultations.

2. **Inform** about potentially difficult moments during testimony.

3. **Anticipate** potential problems in the consultation process.

4. **Discuss** potential early and later conflicts with counsel."[5]

Table 1.2 describes a number of aphorisms and caveats that occur at the "engagement" stage—the earliest phase of the FMHP consultation. At this stage, introductions (or re-introductions) are made; the proposed consultation is discussed; ground rules are set; the agendas and advocacy positions of the consultee (i.e., the retaining attorney or court) and consultant (i.e., the FMHP) are established; business aspects (including financial parameters and time frames) of the consultation are agreed upon and are set; and the FMHP consultation formally begins once a retainer payment is made and received (or agreed upon and documented, in public sector consultations). Aphorisms, caveats, and agendas applicable to the FHMP consultant or "expert" are depicted in the left-hand column, and those of the consultee attorney or court are depicted in the right-hand column.

---

4   *Merriam-Webster Dictionary*. (2016). Merriam-Webster, Inc. Springfield, MA.
5   Greenfield, D. P., Dougherty, E. J., & Zimmermann, M. L. (2019, March 31). *Aphorisms and caveats* [Paper presentation]. 35th Annual Symposium of the American College of Forensic Psychology. San Diego, CA.

While the number and variety of aphorisms and caveats at this beginning stage of the FMHP consultation may seem large and bewildering, they illustrate and underscore the need on both sides (those of the expert and the attorney) to be aware of only a few salient points in this process. These points include the following:

- an awareness of the nature of the referral process (e.g., "How did you learn about me?" "Doctor, I googled you. Do you do this kind of work?")
- the scope of the consultation (e.g., "What's your time crunch?" "Do you know what kind of expert you want?")
- the need for both sides to have their "eyes wide open" from the beginning (e.g., "If it doesn't smell right, it probably isn't." "An expert who consults for a *pro se* client has a fool for a client and a fool for an expert."
- the need to understand the nature and scope of the consultee (e.g., "Doctor, I need a report confirming my client's [fill in the blank]. Will you do that?" "Doctor, I've only done one of these types of cases before. I hope you can help me!")
- the need to be clear about financial arrangements (e.g., "Don't worry about your fee, Doctor. My client is responsible for it, not me.")
- an awareness of and agreement upon a myriad of other points and details at the beginning of this confusing and complicated FMHP consultation process

TABLE 1.2   Engagement

EXPERT	ATTORNEY
• "The lawyer's been awfully busy, and simply didn't have time to discuss the case with you. Will you do the evaluation without speaking with them? Is that all right with you? I hope you don't mind."	• "Use the treating doctor as an expert: They know your client better than an expert does."
• "What's your time crunch?"	• "Doctor, you're the only one who can do this! Nobody else is available. *Please!*"
• "When will you need a written report from me?	• "Doctor, my client doesn't have a lot of money, the case is old, and the court wants to resolve it quickly, in about two to three weeks. Will you help?"
• In general, *Lasciate ogni speranza, voi ch'entrata*. ("Abandon all hope, ye who enter here.")	
• "Do you know what kind of expert you want?"	• "Always wait until the last possible minute to get your expert. After all, you may not need one."
• "How did you learn about me?" "Who referred you to me?"	• "Doctor, I need a report confirming my client's [fill in the blank]. Will you do that?"
• "An individual who represents themselves as a *pro se* client has a fool for a lawyer and a fool for a client." Similarly, "an expert who consults for a *pro se* individual has a fool for a client and a fool for an expert."	• "Doctor, I've only done one of these types of cases before. I hope you can help me, tell me what to do, or advise me. ..." (This is *not* likely to inspire confidence in the expert.)
• The "smell" test: "If it doesn't smell right, it probably isn't."	• "I only want to know my client's exposure, doctor. Only the truth. Nothing else."
• "Attorneys have only one timepiece: the last-minute clock!"	• Letter from counsel to former treating doctor:
• "My lawyer told me I needed an expert, and to find one. I Googled you. Do you do this kind of work?"	"Dear Doctor: Please be advised that the trial for your *patient* is scheduled for three weeks from now, and your testimony will be required. Please advise this office as to your availability."
• For the prospective expert, *caveat emptor* translates to "Know the attorney(s) who is (who are) retaining you."	
• "Certain things don't change: Live with it!"	

In this author's view, the potential for misunderstanding and "deal-break-ing" when you collect your fees during the FMHP consultation process is so great that the aphorisms and caveats for this phase warrant their own table (see Table 1.3, "Collecting Your Fees," below).

TABLE 1.3   Collecting Your Fees

EXPERT	ATTORNEY
▪ *"Do not* wait until the case is over: Retainer! Retainer! Retainer!"	▪ "Doctor, you'll be paid by the insurance company. Your financial relationship is with that company, not with this firm."
	▪ "Don't worry about the expert fee doctor. My client is responsible for it, not me."
	▪ "Doctor, I know my client hasn't paid the balance of your fee. But I have to serve your report *tomorrow*. Please!"

Table 1.4, "Desiderata," (below) gives a list of desirable elements for the FMHP consultant in working with retaining counsel and a court, which should be agreed upon by both consultant and consultee during the engagement stage of the FMHP process.

TABLE 1.4   Desiderata

In an "ideal world," necessary elements for an optimal FMHP consultation referral include the following:

1. A clear consultation request, (or a clear indication that the referral question needs discussion)

2. Adequate lead time (weeks, not days) for the consultation (including records review; interview/examination; preparation of reports; and testimony)

3. *All* available and requested records and materials in *all* available formats (written; DVD; videotapes, etc.) received in a timely and organized fashion, *or* received in sufficient time for the consultant to organize the materials

4. Telephone availability of counsel to discuss the forensic consultations, as needed

5. Clear understanding and satisfaction of consultant's financial requirements by retaining counsel

Finally, Table 1.5, "Rules of Conduct in the Legal Arena for Lawyers and Their Experts," (below) gives a tongue-in-cheek list of undesirable behaviors and foibles by attorneys as sometimes perceived by their clients and experts, which should *not* be practiced by counsel or counsel's expert at any stage of the FMHP consultation process.

TABLE 1.5 Rules of Conduct in the Legal Arena for Lawyers and Their Experts[6]

Inevitably, we and our patients may find ourselves in the legal arena, for one reason or another. Over the years, we have experienced a number of frustrating complaints and developed survival tips for working with counsel.

For example, we should all be aware that many attorneys always abide by the following maxims:

1. *Always* be (or appear to be) harassed and busy.
2. *Never* take responsibility for delays, continuances, adjournments, etc. (*Always* blame the judge or the other side).
3. *Always* pass the responsibility to pay bills on to someone else. ... *Anyone* else.
4. "The check (report, letter, affidavit, memorandum, etc.) is in the mail."
5. "Don't call me—I'll call you."
6. "Forget about it, and it'll go away."
7. *Never* stay in contact with your experts on an ongoing basis.
8. *Always* leap from crisis to crisis:
   a. Corollary: *Always* be in a tearing rush.
   b. Corollary: *Never* do important work until the night before the event.

Professional telephone etiquette is *not* important. (FYI: this can make or break a practice—theirs or yours.)

9. *Do not* assess or use the lawyer's/expert's preferred mode of communication (phone, text, email, USPS/snail mail, smoke signals, etc.).

Do not endorse or use any of the preceding "Rules of Conduct." If you do, your practice will suffer, and likely fail.

Given all these potential landmines—even at this earliest stage of the FMHP consultation process—if this stage is handled satisfactorily and well by both retaining counsel or the court and the expert, both can proceed to the next stage of the process (preparation). They can confidently avoid Dante's wise but chilling advice to *lasciate ogni speranza, voi ch'entrata* ("Abandon all hope, ye who enter here").

---

6   Adapted from Greenfield, D. P. (1999). A modest proposal. *Addiction Insight*, 1(1), 1, 3.

CHAPTER 2

Preparation

"In sex, therapy, business, and life in
general, preparation is everything."

S O, YOU AND counsel have agreed on the ground rules for your FMHP consultation and you have been engaged to consult in this matter. Now you prepare, the next step in the FMHP consultation process.

Table 2.1, "Preparation," presents several aphorisms and caveats encountered by this author over the years, which illustrate both "do's" (e.g., "If it isn't written down, it didn't happen: Document! Document! Document!") and "don'ts" (e.g., "Doctor, I'll send you what I think you'll need in the way of records and materials to review for your report [evaluation].") for counsel and their FMHP consultants. The aphorisms and caveats speak for themselves.

TABLE 2.1 Preparation

EXPERT	ATTORNEY
• "As in therapy, sex, and life in general, preparation is everything."	• "Doctor, I'll send you what I think you'll need in the way of records and materials to review for your report [evaluation]."
• "If it isn't written down, it didn't happen: Document! Document! Document!"	• "Never communicate with your expert, and never, never, *never* return your expert's phone calls, emails, texts, mail, smoke signals, and the like." (See Table 1.5 in Chapter 1.)
• "Create your own authority" by making presentations and writing articles about things that you *do want to do* and *should do*, and about things you *do not want to do* and *should not do*.	• "I don't need to speak with the doctor about the evaluation. They are an experienced litigation consultant and expert witness, and they know what we need from their consultation."
• On advocacy: "Be truthful, but helpful." NO, the FMHC's advocacy is for the truth.	• In a voicemail message (with no prior mention being made of it): "Doctor, this is 'X' from attorney 'Y's' office. Don't forget that your testimony is set for this Thursday, the day after tomorrow. Please be at the courthouse at 8:30 a.m. sharp!"
• On advocacy: Withholding or limiting discovery or other information. NO, the FMHC's advocacy is for the truth.	

Although from a strictly business perspective, conserving costs and reducing expenses may be appealing to counsel (e.g., "Use the treating doctor as an expert: They know your client better than any expert does." "I don't need to speak with the doctor about the evaluation. They are an experienced litigation consultant and expert witness and they know what we need from their consultation."), such a practice on its surface flies in the face of the traditional litigation wisdom that "preparation is everything."

In this author's experience, for example, skimping on obtaining and providing discovery records and materials to the FMHP experts and spending insufficient time, effort, and money preparing the FMHP consultant at any phase of the litigation are unwise practices, which run the risk of the consultant's being unprepared or ill-prepared for whatever might come up (e.g., at testimony and cross-examination).

Despite how collegial and productive the interactions between the retaining counsel and the FMHP expert may be, the core advocacy positions of each are different: Counsel's advocacy position is *for* their client, whereas the FMHP consultant's advocacy position is for their professional opinion *about* counsel's client. That opinion refers to the consultant's response(s) to counsel's question(s) about their client with respect to issues relevant to the case at hand. For example, if counsel requests that the FMHP consultant "be truthful, but helpful", this may raise concerns about the consultant's advocacy, as may "withholding or limiting discovery or other information" from the consultant. As aphorisms and caveats (see Table 2.1), both are noteworthy.

In a very real sense, all the FMHP consultant's professional activities are preparation for further FMHP work. Given the sources and bases of the consultant's expertise and credibility, documentation of that expertise outside the forensic (litigation) context through articles, presentations, teaching, lecturing, and the like also ought to be considered preparation, and from counsel's perspective, it may have implications for the FMHP's expertise and credibility (see Chapter 6, Table 6.2, "Testifying PRN"). For the purposes of this book and to illustrate the above point, several of this author's articles, which illustrate responses to forensic issues and concerns over the years, are given in Table 2.2.

TABLE 2.2   Creating Your Own Authority: The Same Questions Keep Coming Up

	QUESTION/ISSUE	RESPONSE/AUTHORITY
1.	"Doctor, why do the evaluations take so long?"	Greenfield, D. P., San Giacomo, H. L., & Westerkamp, P. (2001). Psychiatric evaluations in employment law. *New Jersey Labor and Employment Law Quarterly, 24*(4): 27–30.
2.	"Doctor, I insist on having copies of all your tests, raw data, and results."	Greenfield, D. P., & McDonough, M. (2000, September/October). Between a rock and a hard place: Ethical and procedural conflicts in providing information in forensic practice. *The Forensic Examiner, 9*(9/10): 16–19.
3.	"Doctor, I'll be sitting in on the examination. I'll be quiet and won't say anything."	Greenfield, D. P. (1999, January/February). Psychiatric/psychological evaluations should not be observed or recorded by opposing counsel. *The Forensic Examiner, 8*(1/2): 23–26.
4.	"Doctor, I insist on knowing the names of the tests you will be giving my client."	Greenfield, D. P., Dougherty, E. J., Podboy, J. W., & Zimmermann, M. L. (2002, April 19). *Three vexing problems in forensic practice* [Paper presentation]. Presentation given at the 18th Annual Symposium of the American College of Forensic Psychology. San Francisco, CA.
5.	"Doctor, I want you to write a report for your patient (who is my client) and testify as an expert for them."	Greenfield, D. P. & Huber, P. (1998, July 27). Should doctors serve as patients' expert witnesses?" *New Jersey Lawyer, 7:* 7.
6.	"Doctor, my client was so drunk, they had a blackout. Doesn't that excuse their behavior?"	Greenfield, D. P., Podboy, J. W., & Zimmermann, M. L. (1999, January). "Blackouts" and amnestic phenomena in the law. *American Journal of Forensic Psychiatry, 20*(1): 19–25.
7.	"Doctor, your report in this matter doesn't follow the usual format for such expert reports, does it?"	Greenfield, D. P. & Gottschalk, J. (2009). *Writing forensic reports: A guide for the mental health professional.* Springer Publishing Company.
8.	"Doctor, what is your diagnosis of this party to this lawsuit? In the final analysis, isn't the diagnosis all that is necessary for your purposes?"	Greenfield, D. P., Zimmermann, M. L., & Dougherty, E. J. (2014). What does psychiatric diagnosis do for the law, anyway? *American Journal of Forensic Psychology, 32*(1): 53–60.

Finally, for preparation purposes, Table 2.3 gives a sample checklist form from the author's practice that summarizes clinical, administrative, and related legal and discovery records and materials generally useful and available for FMHP consultations. In contrast to counsel's plan to "send you what I think you'll need in the way of records and materials to review," this checklist can be completed and supplemented by the expert and given to retaining counsel as a guide to discovery and related records and materials to be obtained for the consultant expert's review in the matter at hand.

The next stage in the FMHP's consultation in the present nine-stage system is the interview/examination (real or virtual) of counsel's client.[1] The interview/examination is only carried out when it is possible, and it does not occur in cases in which a review of records is conducted instead (for example, when a will contest is evaluated). The interview/examination stage will be discussed next, in Chapter 3.

---

1 During the 2020 COVID-19 pandemic—when this book was written—real, live, and face-to-face (the terms are used interchangeably) forensic interviews/examinations were rarely done because of quarantine restrictions. The principles and goals for both real and virtual interviews/examinations, to my understanding, are the same, and both are applicable for present purposes. Additionally, the distinction between real and virtual is irrelevant for forensic evaluation not involving interviews/examinations.

TABLE 2.3 Sample Checklist for Requesting Records and Materials for Review by FMHP Consultant

DANIEL P. GREENFIELD, MD, MPH, MS, FASAM
General Psychiatry • Forensic Psychiatry • Addiction Medicine
62 Old Short Hills Road • Short Hills, New Jersey 07078-2152 • (973) 376-0026 • Fax (973) 376-1196
dpgreenfieldmdpsychiatry@msn.com

Date: _____ RE: _____

Dear _____:

Confirming our recent discussion about the above-referenced matter, below is a completed checklist of the records and materials, which I request you make available for me to review in connection with my evaluation in the above-referenced matter, prior to my actual interview/examination. Please advise me if you have questions about this list, or if you require anything additional from me in connection with this request. Thank you very much.

Sincerely,

Daniel P. Greenfield, MD, MPH, MS, FASAM

Diplomate, American Board of Psychiatry and Neurology (P)
Diplomate, American Board of Addiction Medicine

Medical Records and Materials
- Hospital records (notes, test results, laboratory data, order sheets, nursing notes, etc.)

- Outpatient records (notes, test results, laboratory tests, etc.)

- Consultations (clinical evaluation/ treatment)

- Reports (evaluations, forensic records, independent medical examinations [IMEs])

- Testing records and materials (psychological and related)

- Prior hospital, medical, outpatient, etc., records (unrelated to the case)

- Supplemental Security Income (SSI)/ Disability Determination Services (DDS) records/files

- Other:

Administrative/Legal Records and Materials
- *All* criminal/legal/discovery records (includes police reports, investigation reports, supplemental reports, autopsy reports, evidence records, toxicology/pathology reports, etc.)

- *All* complaints (initial, amended, etc.)

- *All* replies to complaints

- *All* interrogatories and answers to interrogatories

- Deposition transcripts and summaries

- Employment/personnel records

- Prior employment/personnel records

- *All* school records (including Child Study Team records and reports, if applicable)

- Prior legal/case records and materials

- Other:

CHAPTER 3

The Interview/Examination

"Doctor, I'll be sitting in on your interview.
Don't worry, I won't interfere. I'll be quiet as a mouse."

As in clinical/therapeutic practice, a core feature of an FMHP consultation is the face-to-face (or virtual; see Chapter 2) interview/examination in which "the basic parameters and milieu of an independent medical examination (IME) are essentially the same as for a clinical interview or session: privacy, quiet, non-interference from others, and an environment in which information and ideas can be freely exchanged" (Greenfield, 1999).

Now, no reader of this book would be so naïve as to think that the skeptical FMHP consultant would accept the above idealized statement or that both the FMHP consultant—whose advocacy position is *not* for retaining counsel's client (see above, Chapter 1)—and counsel would be completely unbiased with respect to their respective advocacy and agenda. However, to the extent that such idealized conditions can be achieved, in the interest of unbiased information, all involved in this process—counsel, the FMHP consultant, and the court—should attempt to achieve them.

In this author's experience, Table 3.1 presents two common scenarios in which counsel seeks to influence the conditions of the FMHP consultant's interview/examination of counsel's client. Table 3.2 lists four articles by this author and others that counter those efforts by counsel. As a practical matter, the extent to which FMHP consultations/evaluations are influenced by counsel, in this author's experience, are largely determined by law. Therefore, an FMHP consultant's interview/examination, as an exercise and effort based on clinical science, should attempt to maintain the sanctity of clinical science as much as possible.

TABLE 3.1 The Interview/Examination

ATTORNEY

"Doctor, I'll be sitting in on your interview. Don't worry, I won't interfere. I'll be as quiet as a mouse."

"Doctor, why does your interview take so long? Other doctors do these interviews in about 15 minutes."

TABLE 3.2 Create Your Own Authority

ATTORNEY

Greenfield, D. P. (1999, January/February). Psychiatric/psychological examinations should not be observed or recorded by opposing counsel. *The Forensic Examiner*, 8(1/2): 23–27.

Greenfield, D. P. (2001). Psychiatric evaluations. *New Jersey Labor & Employment Law Quarterly*, 24(1): 31.

Greenfield, D. P. & McDonough, M. (2000, September/October). Between a rock and a hard place. *The Forensic Examiner*, 9(9/10): 16–19.

Greenfield, D. P., SanGiacomo, H. & Westerkamp, P. (2001). Psychiatric evaluations in employment law. *New Jersey Labor & Employment Law Quarterly*, 24(1): 27–30.

CHAPTER 4

Collecting Your Thoughts

"Don't you want to know my opinion
before you get my report?"

I N THE HISTORY of science, the Elizabethan Englishman Francis Bacon (1561–1626)—a lawyer and government official by training and profession—was known as an early user of what subsequently came to be refined as "the scientific method:" He was a gatherer, collector, coordinator, and reporter of information.[1]

The analogy for this book is that as an FMHP consultant, Bacon would have accumulated data and synthesized it into a forensic mental health report responsive to the questions, issues, and concerns that he had been asked to address. Analogous to scientific reporting, he collected his thoughts, took the time and effort for his data and impressions to rumble around and consolidate in his brain, and then formulated it into a responsive report.

---

1   Without belaboring the point, it remained for later thinkers to refine Bacon's early method of collecting and organizing data—the "pre-scientific method"—by incorporating hypothesis formation and testing into the scientific method. In this vein, a later work of Bertrand Russell (Russell, B. [1959]. *Wisdom of the west*. Doubleday & Company, Inc. New York, NY.) stated the following: "But as to the formulation of hypotheses, Bacon is wrong in thinking that this is based on induction, which is concerned rather with the testing of hypotheses. Indeed, in order to conduct a series of observations one already has to have a preliminary hypothesis. But for the discovery of hypotheses, one cannot lay down a set of general prescriptions. Bacon is quite wrong in thinking that there could be an instrument of discovery, the mechanical application of which would enable one to unearth startling new secrets of nature. The setting up of hypotheses does not proceed in this manner at all. Again, Bacon's rejection of the syllogism led him to underestimate the function of deduction in scientific enquiry. In particular, he had little appreciation of the mathematical methods which were developing in his time. The role of induction in this testing of hypotheses is one small facet of method. Without the mathematical deduction which leads from the hypotheses to a concrete, testable situation, there would be no knowing what to test" (p. 191).

Table 4.1 gives four aphorisms and caveats, which illustrate the need for the FMHP consultant to "collect their thoughts," and reason in such a way as to develop a logical, coherent, and science-based formulation of their expert opinion, consistent with and taking into account legal definitions and requirements, and responsive to the legal questions, issues, and concerns to be addressed in the FMHP consultation at hand. This is a tall order, failures and shortcomings of which are illustrated in Table 4.1, and which will be discussed below.

TABLE 4.1   Collecting Your Thoughts

EXPERT	ATTORNEY
■ "I'm an advocate for my expert opinion in this matter, not for either side." ■ "Don't you want to know my opinion before you get my report?" ■ "Are there really laws of nature, or do we believe in them only because of our own innate love of order?" —Russell, B. (1945). *A history of western philosophy*, p. xi.	■ "But doctor, my client has a diagnosis of schizophrenia. She must have been insane when she killed her landlady." (psychosis ≠ legal insanity) ■ "But doctor, my client had a blackout during the incident. He couldn't be criminally responsible for killing his partner."

I'm an advocate for my expert opinion in
this matter, not for either side.
—Greenfield & Huber (1998)[2]

This point recurs often in the nine stages of the FMHP consultation process. It emphasizes the advocacy position of the expert and should discourage retaining counsel from attempting to sway the consultant away from their advocacy position. Another aphorism previously discussed—"be truthful, but helpful"—applies to representing counsel, not to the opining expert.

"Don't you want to know my opinion before you get my report?"

This frequent question of the FMHP consultant, usually asked very shortly after the conclusion of the expert's interview/examination with retaining counsel, illustrates the different advocacy positions and agendas of counsel and the FMHP consultant. In their own mind, counsel "needs a report confirming my client's [fill in the blank]" (see Table 1.2). Therefore, the objective

---

2   Greenfield, D. P., & Huber, H. (1998, July). *Should doctors serve as patients' expert witnesses.* New Jersey Lawyer 7(7): 17–18.

of the consultant's work from counsel's perspective is to obtain that report as soon as possible (especially in view of attorneys' tendencies to delay, postpone, and otherwise put off expert activities as long as possible; this is part of the "last-minute clock" tactic, see Table 1.2). The FMHP consultant's objective, on the other hand, is to provide an evidence-based clinically scientific opinion (and a report if, in the final analysis, counsel wants such a report). From a cognitive perspective, this process requires time for analyzing and processing the data and then developing an opinion. Before the expert memorializes that opinion, counsel should know what it is.

> *Are there really laws of nature, or do we believe in them*
> *only because of our own innate love of order?*
> —Bertrand Russell (1945)[3]

This quote refers to a central cognitive task of the FMHP consultant in organizing information and data (obtained from a variety of sources) about the lawyer's client to offer a response (an expert forensic opinion) to counsel's or the court's questions and concerns. This task boils down to inferences and constructs about an evaluee's underlying mental state and psychiatric or neuropsychiatric condition to address questions of criminal responsibility (in criminal cases), of effects of exposures and experiences (in civil matters), and of divorce and child custody questions (in family law). In addressing such legal concerns and questions, the FMHP consultant must take into account legal constructs and concepts as well as clinical science constructs and concepts and make them "fit" together to the extent that they do. These comments do not respond to Russell's query, but they do support the need for the FMHP consultant to "collect their thoughts" in arriving at a responsive opinion for their consultation.

> *"But doctor, my client has a diagnosis of schizophrenia.*
> *She **must** have been insane when she killed her*
> *landlady." (psychosis ≠ legal insanity)*

The frustrated attorney in the above quote (1) conflated "psychosis," or "diagnosis" (a clinical concept) with "legal insanity" (a legal concept); and (2) demonstrated the differences in advocacy and agenda between attorneys and their FMHP consultants. Without belaboring these points, in a paper entitled "What Does Psychiatric Diagnosis Do for the Law, Anyway?" Greenfield et al. (2014) first wrote that "To reify a 'diagnosis' and empower it with some sort

---

3   Russell, B. (1945). *A history of western philosophy.* Simon and Schuster/Touchstone. New York, NY. Page xi.

of legal decisional power it simply does not have ... is wrong. ..."[4] The authors further explained that "the application of concepts of 'diagnosis' by the law in forensic psychiatric and psychological concepts tends to make two errors, known in research methodology as 'Type I' (attributing a feature or characteristic to an entity which it does not have. This is also known in epidemiology as a 'false positive,' and more generally as an 'error of commission') and 'Type II' (not attributing a feature or characteristic to an entity which it does have. This is also known in epidemiology as a 'false negative,' and more generally as an 'error of omission'). ..."[5] In the comment made by frustrated counsel above about the client with a diagnosis of schizophrenia, a Type I error is made by counsel in attributing a legal status ("legally insane") to a clinical diagnosis ("schizophrenia"). "[T]he attorney, in essence, asserts 'This defendant has a diagnosis of schizophrenia, and must be crazy [psychotic] all the time. So, he had to be crazy [psychotic] at the time of the offense, and therefore, not criminally responsible." In summary "what matters is not the underlying **diagnosis**, but the **symptoms** from that diagnosis."[6]

> "But doctor, my client had a blackout during the incident. He couldn't be criminally responsible for killing his partner."

Although the frustrated attorney who attempted to persuade the FMHP consultant about blackouts did not exactly make a Type I or Type II reasoning error, they did equate memory loss (a clinical concept) with lack of criminal responsibility (a criminal/legal concept). As well settled in both clinical science and the law, the term "'blackout' ... carries no particular legal implications ... [and in] ... the absence of a confounding factor, such as epilepsy, the presence of amnesia carries no particular legal implications, and the differentiation of authentic from feigned amnesia may not be critical,"[7] and "the blackout refers only to memory function (or lack thereof) after an event, and not to the nature of the behaviors during the event."[8] With respect to this particular aphorism, from the FMHP consulting expert's perspective as well as from counsel's, the aphorism is wrong. Don't bother!

---

4   Greenfield, D. P., Zimmerman, M. L., & Dougherty, E. J. (2014). What does psychiatric diagnosis do for the law, anyway? *American Journal of Forensic Psychology, 32*(1): 53–60.
5   Greenfield, D. P., Zimmerman, M. L., & Dougherty, E. J. (2014). What does psychiatric diagnosis do for the law, anyway? *American Journal of Forensic Psychology, 32*(1): 53–60.
6   Greenfield, D. P., Podboy, J. W., & Zimmermann, M. L. (1999). "Blackouts" and amnestic phenomena in the law. *American Journal of Forensic Psychiatry, 20*(1): 19–25.
7   Kopelman, H. D. (1987). Crime and amnesia: review. *Behavioral Science and the Law, 5*(3): 313–392.
8   Ibid.

After the FMHP consultant has collected their thoughts, the next stage in the consultation/evaluation process—the fifth step—is that of report preparation (if counsel or the court wants a report; see above: "Don't you want to know my opinion before you get my report?").

The aphorisms and caveats for that step follow in Chapter 5.

The Report

Usually, the first comprehensive exposure a lawyer or judge will have to an expert's opinion is through his or her report.
—Dickinson R. Debevoise, U.S. District Judge (2009)

"Nobody ever reads these things anyway, except my [mother, father, partner, wife, lover, children ...]."

"Within the four corners of the report ..."

"Doctor, your report doesn't comply with the required formats for such reports, does it?"

I N THE FIRST chapter of *Writing Forensic Reports: A Guide for Mental Health Professionals*, Greenfield and Gottshalk wrote:

> In forensic (unlike clinical) mental health practice, one of the two main products created is the report containing the evaluation of the individual or topic on whom or on which the legal case is based. The other product—not nearly as common as the written report—is live or videotaped testimony at trial, hearing, or deposition.

> "The evaluation (forensic) mental health professional ... must generally prepare a written opinion report about the forensic psychiatric/neuropsychiatric/addiction medicine/other issues involved in the case evaluation. That report is a critical and primary element in terms of the forensic practitioner's participation in the case. By contrast, for the clinical surgeon, for example, the operative report and hospital discharge summary are secondary to the surgical procedure and treatment themselves. These reports are necessary for documentation,

statistical, and medicolegal purposes, and ... are often considered a necessary evil by most surgeons who must prepare them ...[1]

Since the advocacy position of counsel and counsel's (but not the court's[2]) FMHP consultant are different, counsel will usually decide if they want a written opinion report from the consultant (hence, "Don't you want to know my opinion before you get my report?") for the case at hand.[3]

When counsel does want a written report, what should that report look like? The report should be clear, succinct but comprehensive, responsive to counsel's or the court's questions, useful as a guide or road map to testimony (see Chapter 6, "Testifying PRN"), and otherwise adherent to the guidelines in *Writing Forensic Reports* (Greenfield and Gottshalk [2008]). Notwithstanding the periodically heard aphorism that such reports are not actually (or fully, or carefully) read, when counsel or the court wants a report, or is confronted by one, the report *is* read and used. With such a "performative"—(performing the task of persuading those involved of the FMHP expert's opinion[4])—report, clear and concise writing is essential. The Appendix to this present chapter presents excerpts from what, in this author's view, is among the best short pieces about that topic; the excerpts come from George Orwell's essay entitled "Politics and the English Language" (1946).

With any report, a number of aphorisms and caveats may apply. These are given in Table 5.1 (below).

---

1   Greenfield, D. P., and Gottshalk, J. A. (2008). The importance of forensic reports. In *Writing forensic reports: A guide for mental health professionals*, Springer Publishing Co. New York, NY. p. 3. Aphorisms and caveats concerning testimony are discussed in this book in Chapter 6 ("Testifying PRN") and Chapter 7 ("On Cross-Examination").

2   Interestingly, since the FMHP expert's task is to provide the truth with respect to the questions and issues presented, and the court's task is to determine the truth of these issues and balance the rights of the parties with respect to these questions and issues, the advocacy positions of the consultant/expert may well turn out to be similar to those of the court. This point is discussed in many legal and FMHP writings, and is well beyond the scope of this present volume.

3   Ibid. p. 3. As a practical matter, the significant exception to this general proposition occurs when an FMHP consultant for the prosecution offers a mitigating or exculpatory opinion to the prosecuting consultee. To my understanding, since the duty of the prosecution—the state—is to provide exculpatory as well as inculpatory evidence to the court, the prosecution is obligated to provide an adverse (to the prosecution) expert opinion and report to the court, even if the expert opinion does not support the prosecution's theory of the case. This is also a point about which considerable writing and discussion may be found, also well beyond the scope of this present volume.

4   Griffin, E. (2007). The place of performative writing in forensic psychiatry. *The Journal of the American Academy of Psychiatry and the Law*, 35(1), 27–31.

TABLE 5.1 The Report

EXPERT	ATTORNEY
▪ "Nobody ever reads these things anyway, except my [mother, father, partner, husband, wife, lover, children ...]."	▪ "Doctor, your report doesn't comply with the required formats for such reports, does it?"
▪ "Don't you want to know my opinion before you get my report?"	▪ "Within the four corners of the report ..."
▪ "There's no one happier than a lawyer who receives an expert's report on time, or even early."	▪ "I promise you, Doctor, your report is a work product. Drafts are not discoverable."
	▪ "Doctor, your report is fine. There are a few changes that will help, but I'll make them myself and serve your report on opposing counsel. I don't want to trouble you. ..."
	▪ "Doctor, your report's late. Where is it? The court wants it!"

Timing and meeting deadlines can be stressful in the context of reports (when counsel requires a written report). The aphorisms and caveats from Table 5.1 apply in this context, namely that

1. "There's no one happier than a lawyer who receives an expert's report on time, or even early."

2. "Doctor, your report is fine. There are a few changes that will help, but I'll make them myself and serve your report on opposing counsel. I don't want to trouble you." (This is **definitely** not advisable!)

3. "Doctor, your report's late. Where is it? The court wants it!"

The first aphorism speaks for itself. However, the second aphorism (even if the helpful attorney's editing might actually save time) is inadvisable for a number of self-evident reasons, not the least of which is that with the attorney's editing, the report ceases to be solely the FMHP consultant/expert's report. Aside from the dishonesty of that situation, should it occur and be discovered (e.g., during testimony), the value of the report and expert's opinion could at the very least be compromised, and at worst be invalidated. In any event, that situation could seriously damage the case and the FMHP consultant's reputation, and the practice should not be allowed.

The third aphorism may stem from a number of reasons, including an outstanding bill due to the FMHP consultant/expert. While financial requirements (see Table 1.2, "Engagement") should in theory prevent misunderstandings of this type, and while the FMHP consultant/expert may be correct in refusing to provide services if financial requirements are not met by counsel,[5] the pressure of court deadlines, in my experience, may make it difficult for the FMHP consultant/expert not to comply with counsel's demands for reports and related services when counsel places the "blame," or demand, on the court. From the FMHP consultant/expert's perspective, this situation will periodically happen: "Live with it!"

Concerning the nature, structure, and extent of the report, the aphorisms and caveats that apply (see Table 5.1) are the following:

1. "Doctor, your report doesn't comply with the required formats for such expert reports, does it?"

2. "Within the four corners of the report ..."

3. "I promise you, Doctor, your report is a work product. Drafts are not discoverable."

The first aphorism was the impetus for the writing of *Writing Forensic Reports* (see Selected References on p. xvi) and allowed the authors to find out that at the time, no specific "required format" existed for forensic reports.[6] As a baiting question of the FMHP consultant/expert, for example at deposition, the expert should respond to the inaccuracy in response to the question (e.g., "There is no 'required format' for such reports."). These points are discussed further in Chapter 6 ("Testifying PRN") and Chapter 7 ("On Cross-Examination").

"Within the four corners of the report" refers to the completeness of the FMHP consultant/expert's report and the concept that all of the expert's information and opinions should be memorialized or referenced in the written report. As a practical matter, however, in this writer's experience, "wide latitude" (a term of art in sworn testimony) is usually given to such expert testimony, often permitting expansion during testimony of points not explicitly made in writing in the report (Expert: "It's not written in my report in so many words, but I'm testifying about it now. ...")

---

5 The FMHP consultant/expert has a financial relationship with counsel, and not with counsel's client or the insurance company of counsel's client. See Table 1.2, "Engagement."

6 At the time, minimal requirements for the content of expert reports were articulated in the law (see U.S. Code, Title V, Rule 26—Duty to Disclose in the 2019 *Federal Rules of Civil Procedure*) and there were few guidelines suggested in the forensic literature.

Last, as a practical matter, although it is not the FMHP consultant/expert's "job" to know applicable substantive and procedural law concerning such questions as whether drafts of a report constitute "work product" (and are not discoverable, or not fully discoverable), it behooves the expert to ask such questions of retaining counsel (or the court), learn the answer, and respond accordingly. The expert's reputation may ride on that response.

A last point in the context of FMHP consultations and evaluations is addressed by the question "What Does Psychiatric Diagnosis Do for the Law, Anyway?," as discussed above.[7] In criminal law cases, for example, questions of criminal responsibility may be determined by the existence of an underlying potentially mitigating or exculpatory "mental disease or deficit," worded in different ways in different jurisdictions. In Greenfield et al. (2014), the authors point out that a diagnosis does not equate to a "mental disease or deficit"; for that reason, we do not emphasize "psychiatric diagnosis" in our reports.

In the next step of the nine-step process, the FMPH consultant/expert's report has been written and accepted by counsel (or the court), and negotiations among counsel (or the court) have proceeded. It becomes clear over this period of time that the parties will not settle, and that (first) deposition and (later) hearing/trial sworn testimony will be required to advance the case. The fifth step in this process—"Testifying PRN"—is next, and will be discussed in Chapter 6.

Appendix: Clear and Persuasive Report Writing

One of the best short pieces on clear, concise, and persuasive writing is Orwell's essay, "Politics and the English Language" (1946).[8]

Several particularly powerful excerpts from this essay follow:

> There is a long list of flyblown metaphors which could similarly be got rid of if enough people would interest themselves in the job; and it should be possible to laugh the not "un-" formation out of existence, to reduce the amount of Latin and Greek in the average sentence, to drive out foreign phrases and strayed scientific words, and, in general, to make pretentiousness unfashionable.[9]

---

7   Greenfield, D. P., Zimmermann, M. L., & Dougherty, E. J. (2014). What does psychiatric diagnosis do for the law, anyway? *American Journal of Forensic Psychology*, 32(1): 53–60
8   Orwell, G. (1991). *Down and out in Paris and London; 1984; shooting an elephant and other essays.* Quality Paperback Books. New York, NY. p. 77–92.
9   Ibid. p. 91.

One can cure oneself of the not un- formation by memorizing this sentence: A not unblack dog was chasing a not unsmall rabbit across a not ungreen field.[10]

Orwell provides six situations in which "one needs rules that one can rely on when instinct fails":[11]

- Never use a metaphor, simile, or other figure of speech which you are used to seeing in print.
- Never use a long word when a short one will do.
- If it is possible to cut a word out, always cut it out.
- Never use the passive when you can use the active.
- Never use a foreign phrase, a scientific word, or a jargon word if you can think of an everyday English equivalent.
- Break any of these rules sooner than saying anything outright barbarous.[12]

10　Ibid. p. 90.
11　Ibid. p. 91.
12　Ibid. p. 92.

CHAPTER 6

Testifying PRN[1]

The Scariest Part of the Process

NOT SURPRISINGLY, THE most fear-producing activity among unextraordinary types of activities—excluding such strongly fearful activities as skydiving, rescuing damsels in distress in spy novels, and Navy SEAL activities— is public speaking. Table 6.1 provides a list of fears based on a survey of what people find the scariest. The result is typical among such surveys.

TABLE 6.1   A Few of the Scariest Things[2]

- Spiders—arachnophobia
- Confined spaces—claustrophobia
- **Public speaking—glossophobia**
- Heights—acrophobia
- Zombies—kinemortophobia
- Thunder and Lightning—astraphobia
- The dentist—dentophobia
- Darkness—nyctophobia

---

1   "PRN" from the Latin, *pro re necessitate*, or "as the thing is needed." This term is frequently used in medical practice, for example, for instructions in prescription writing by physicians, dentists, and other such healthcare providers. For present purposes, the title of this chapter suggests that testimony—including expert testimony—does not always occur, except when necessary. In this practitioner's case, for example, notwithstanding my having testified in various hearings, depositions, and/or trials about 15 to 20 times per year for many years, this figure represents the tip of the iceberg in my overall FMHP practice: Only about 8–10% of all forensic cases undertaken per year have gone to a sworn testimony stage. Most cases settle. In my and colleagues' experience, that is a typical percentage in an FMHP practice.

2   Osborn, C. O., & Legg, T. J. (2019) *Common and unique fears explained*. Healthline.com. Healthline Media, Inc. New York, NY. The list in Table 6.1 is excerpted from the list given in the article cited. Retrieved from https://www.healthline.com/health/list-of-phobias on August 14, 2021.

A particularly telling personal example occurred many years ago when a federal-prosecutor-turned-law-professor colleague responded to my comment that participating in a moot court law school exercise as a mock medical expert witness was "kind of fun," and that "maybe I'd like to do more of this in my career." He asked me if I "really wanted to be on public display, humiliated, calumniated, insulted, discredited, and otherwise made to look as stupid and unbelievable as possible for years and years to come?" (He was referring to cross-examination.) I was surprised by this comment, but ended up not taking his implied advice.

As a type of evidence, sworn expert testimony (in hearings, depositions, and trials) by individuals with specialized knowledge and expertise "beyond the ken of the average juror" (or words to that effect) has a long history in the law. As described in a useful article by Dvoskin and Guy (2008), however, the expert witness testimony process is "not about you": The expert's job is to educate, inform, and offer "opinion" (not "fact") evidence for the "trier" or "finder" of fact (i.e., the jury or the court).[3] This may sometimes occur at the cost of the expert's own personal and professional narcissism. The expert witness is part of the litigation process, and by no means a major part, despite what we see on television and in movies, and read in newspapers and novels.

When testimony **is** necessary (PRN), a number of aphorisms and caveats may apply both to counsel and to the FMHP expert. These are described in Table 6.2.

TABLE 6.2 Testifying PRN

EXPERT	ATTORNEY
• "Before, during, and after testimony, go early, go often." —David Flicker, MD, ca. 1990	• "I don't need my own expert. I'll cross-examine opposing counsel's expert."
• "As in therapy, sex, and life in general, *timing* is everything."	• "I have a good, experienced expert. They don't need much preparation."
• "Be prepared for unprepared direct examination *and* cross-examination, including irrelevant and unanswerable questions."	• "We'll have you in and out [in an hour/very quickly], Doctor. Don't worry about your schedule."
• "Never underestimate opposing counsel."	

---

3   Dvoskin, J., & Guy, L. (2008) On being an expert witness: It's not about you. *Psychiatry, Psychology and Law,* 15(2): 202–212.

Like much of forensic practice, several of these aphorisms have to do with timing and scheduling. Specifically, "As in therapy, sex, and life in general, *timing* is everything" is a truism that does not need elaboration. On the other hand, "We'll have you in and out [in an hour/very quickly], Doctor. Don't worry about your schedule," in my experience, is a phrase much more honored in the breach than in practice: As a practical matter, attorneys and the court have almost no control over timing and scheduling in court proceedings, so that—in the prophetic words of a psychologist colleague many years ago—"Things take longer than they do." The astute and experienced FMHP expert should not overschedule: It is an exercise in futility!

The remaining aphorisms in Table 6.2 pertain to preparation, which an experienced and effective trial attorney once told me is "98.6% of the battle." (She never told me what the remaining 1.4% was.) "Before, during, and after testimony, go early, go often" (a riff on the admonition to "Vote early, vote often" in the glory days of early 20th-century Jersey City politics) obviously refers to the expert's feeling physically comfortable during testimony. If the expert feels sick, they should not testify, regardless of the repercussions for the court's schedule. Potentially, the expert's credibility, their reputation, and the outcome of the case could all be at stake with an unhealthy testifying expert.

From counsel's perspective, the aphorism "I don't need my own expert. I'll cross-examine opposing counsel's expert" is obviously a judgment call for counsel. However, having decided to retain an expert in a case that eventually goes to trial (or deposition or hearing), counsel's aphorism that "I have a good, experienced expert. They don't need much preparation" could not be more wrong, in my view. While an experienced expert who has a good working relationship with retaining counsel can save time in preparation for testimony, the nuances of testimony and the benefits of a practice or rehearsal should not be discounted; they should be carried out: "Preparation is 98.6% of the battle."

Now, sometimes direct examining and/or cross-examining counsel is not as prepared as the FMHP expert, and the aphorism for the expert to "Be prepared for unprepared direct examination *and* cross-examination, including irrelevant and unanswerable questions" holds true. For the testifying expert, this situation is an unexpected boon, but not one the expert can count on: Luck is one thing, but nothing substitutes for thorough preparation. The FMHP expert should not underestimate opposing counsel and should insist on preparation from retaining counsel!

Once testimony begins, allowing for the vicissitudes and convenience of the court, it continues to its conclusion.[4] In this author's experience, generally only two events can disrupt or interrupt testimony with a deferment, postponement, adjournment, continuance, or the like: scheduled vacations (for counsel or members the court, but not for the expert witness) or death.

In addition to the substance of the FMHP's testimony, several nuanced expressions that come up repeatedly in testimony should be familiar to the FMHP expert. These have to do with the confidence of the testifying expert in their opinion and the time frame of the opinion.

Concerning the former, "reasonable medical probability," "reasonable medical certainty," and "reasonable medical probability/certainty" or (RMP, RMC, and RMP/C) correspond to the legal concept of the "standard of proof" in civil cases of "more likely than not," also known as "preponderance of the evidence." Although the FMHP expert may be offering an opinion about a matter requiring a different *legal* standard for resolving the case (e.g., "clear and convincing evidence" for resolving such mental health law cases as civil commitment/involuntary hospitalization of reportedly dangerous, seriously mentally ill individuals: about 75% confidence), the FMHP expert's opinion is offered at the level of "more likely than not," or $\geq 50\%$ confidence.

Another nuanced expression with which the FMHP expert witness should be familiar has to do with time frames of legal matters. In that context, Table 6.3 gives an overview of time frames applicable in FMHP evaluation in criminal and quasi-criminal cases. Reference is made in this table to the concept of "reasonably foreseeable future," or consensus reached by a group of superior court judges in New Jersey in 2006; this consensus is described in the footnote in Table 6.3.

---

4   The word *testimony* has an interesting etymology. From the Latin *testis* (singular), *testes* (plural) meaning both "witness" or "spectator," and "testicle." Folklore has it that the former comes from the assumption that in ancient Rome when two men were taking an oath in a public forum, in order to express their truthfulness, they held and swore upon their testes. Presumably, if one broke the oath, his testes would have been lopped off. However, the historical and fossil records provide no written confirmation of that practice, to this author's knowledge.

TABLE 6.3   Time Frames for Criminal and Quasi-Criminal Psychiatric Evaluations

PAST	PRESENT	FUTURE*
At time of investigation	**Competency to stand trial/ proceed to trial**	**Dangerousness**
Legal Insanity	Civil commitment (present dangerousness)	Civil commitment (involuntary psychiatric hospitalization)
Diminished capacity	Sex offenders	Sexual civil commitment (sexually violent predator [SVP]/ sexually dangerous person [SPD])
Intoxication	Civil commitment (involuntary hospitalization)	Outpatient registration of sex offenders ("Megan's Law")
Other commitments		Outpatient civil commitment ("Kendra's Law" in New York)

At time of offense

Miranda rights waiver

For the "reasonably foreseeable future." An unpublished consensus among 35 superior court judges in New Jersey, from an internal poll conducted on November 21, 2006, agreed with a time frame of weeks to months—in contrast to other time frames such as days to weeks, or months to years—for this standard of "reasonably foreseeable future."[5] This author, the 35 polled superior court judges, and numerous other research services do not define a more specific time frame for this standard.

---

5   Data derived from an informal show-of-hands survey taken by this author during the author's lecture to the judges on November 21, 2006.

Continuing with the nine stages of this book, direct examination testimony is now complete, and will be followed by cross-examination of the testifying FMHP expert witness. This process may be considered an extension of the basic constitutional right of the accused to confront their accuser, during which the cross-examining attorney (representing the opposite party about whom the testifying FMHP expert is testifying) attempts to challenge and at least to neutralize the FMHP expert's testimony. In that vein, an applicable aphorism (see below) to the cross-examiner is:

> *"If you have bad facts, argue the law;*
> *if you have bad law, argue the facts;*
> *if you have bad both, attack the expert."*

On to cross-examination!

CHAPTER 7

On Cross-Examination

This is fun ... kind of!
—R. L. Sadoff, March 2000, personal communication

... Until you get burned, you don't know how hot the fire is.
—L. Wright, January 4 and 11, 2021
"The Plague Year," *The New Yorker*

T HE LATE ROBERT L. Sadoff, MD, a pioneer forensic psychiatrist and mentor to this author, periodically commented that "Direct examination is scripted and boring. Cross-examination is challenging and fun! I much prefer it."

From the FMHP expert witness's perspective, an effective cross-examination, as described in Chapter 6, is the opportunity for opposing counsel to at least neutralize the testifying FMHP expert, to discredit the expert altogether, or to reduce the impact and effectiveness of the expert, especially in jury trials.

With such a broad and fluid mandate, the cross-examination process is a rich source of aphorisms and caveats for the FMHP expert, as presented in Tables 7.1 and 7.2.

TABLE 7.1   On Cross-Examination

EXPERT	ATTORNEY
▪ Don't be shy. You're the expert, the lawyer isn't.	▪ "Just one or two more questions [minutes], doctor."
▪ Don't argue with the cross-examiner, but hold your position—when reasonable—and be assertive without being aggressive.	▪ "I don't mean to give you a hard time, doctor, *but** ..."
▪ The "down-home professor" presentation works well.	▪ "Now, I'm not an expert like you, doctor, *but** ..."
	* Wonderful word, "but:" It negates everything that precedes it.

TABLE 7.2   On Cross-Examination

ATTORNEY	EXPERT
"Doctor, I want you to list *everything* on which you relied in arriving at your opinion. *Everything!* Don't leave anything out!" [Especially at deposition.]	"Counselor, that's impossible. If by 'relied' you mean I accept everything I've ever learned, read, or known specifically in connection with this evaluation and report, then I relied fully on nothing. If you mean sources of information directly relevant to my opinion in this matter, then those sources are given on pages [ ] to [ ] of my evaluation report of [date] in this matter."

The first three aphorisms in Table 7.1 are from the FHMP expert's perspective and are self-evident: The *raison d'etre* for the expert is *expertise* "beyond the ken of the average juror." Even if the expert does not feel fully comfortable and confident as an expert, it behooves them always to keep in mind that they are the expert, *not* counsel or the court or the jury. If the expert's testimony is deficient, especially in the long term, then market forces will press that FMHP expert out of that line of work. But while testifying, the *expert* is exactly that, and ought to be confident, humble (presenting as a "down-home professor"), assertive (but not aggressive or argumentative), and a strong advocate for their professional opinion.

The next three aphorisms in Table 7.1 are from the cross-examining counsel's perspective, and in my experience, are meant to "soften up" the expert in anticipation of a "zinger" question or line of questions. Experts beware!

As cross-examination continues, counsel will likely look for ways to "attack (discredit) the witness." One timeworn technique for this is illustrated in Table 7.2 by counsel's demand and the responsive and astute FMHP expert's reply. Again, experts beware! Do not be intimidated!

Still another point has to do with winding down and completing cross-examination. The process eventually has to end, ideally without drawn-out, redundant, boring, or unnecessary content provided by either counsel or expert. In that sense, the testifying expert should give brief and direct responses to counsel's questions, allowing for sufficient latitude and discussion for an adequate response:

> **Attorney:** "Doctor, I want you to give simply 'yes' or 'no' answers to my questions. Will you agree to do that?"
>
> **FMHP Expert:** "Yes, Counsel, I will if I can. But sometimes questions require more than a 'yes' or 'no' response to be accurate, truthful, and responsive. In those instances, I will not restrict my responses to a simple 'yes' or 'no.'"

Generally speaking, cross-examination expert responses should be brief, when possible, especially toward the end of the often tedious and draining process of cross-examination.

Finally, from the cross-examining counsel's perspective, the process has to end somehow. The long-held practices of discontinuing either a long and fruitless cross-examination ("cut your losses") or discontinuing a long but fruitful cross-examination are illustrated by these aphorisms and caveats:

- "If it ain't broke, don't fix it!"
- "Leave well enough alone!"
- "Let it be!"

And in that vein, the admonition to counsel *not* to "ask that last question" is analogous to the skiing admonition not to "take the last ski run of the day." The admonition is well illustrated by the following apocryphal folktale about Vincent Van Gogh:

> **Counsel:** "How do you know he bit off his ear?"
> **Witness:** "I saw him spit it out!"

CHAPTER 8

Collecting Your Fees

*The most successful, respected, and admired forensic
experts ... strive ... to explain their opinion as clearly
as possible ... this stance ... allows one to practice
successfully, over time, in a manner that is as lucrative
as it is ethical. Not bad work if you can get it.*
—Dvoskin and Guy (2008)[1]

A S DESCRIBED IN the Preface, this book's main intended audience is the FMHP in independent practice. For that person, collecting fees is such an important aspect of the practice that it bears repeating (from Chapter 1, "Engagement") and elaborating.

Some models of forensic mental health consulting involve employed mental health professionals—such as staff members of state and county mental hospitals and court liaison mental health professionals—who do not have to rely on earned income from their forensic consulting activities. Such professionals will not need to be concerned about collecting fees.[2]

For the rest of us, however, the aphorisms and caveats discussed in this chapter are important to the viability of our practices, especially collecting our fees. Attention, focus, and follow-up to financial aspects of our

---

1   Dvoskin, J., & Guy, L. (2008) "On being an expert witness: It's not about you." *Psychiatry, Psychology and Law,* 15(2), p. 202–212.

2   Generally, it is inadvisable for the consulting and treating FHMP for any given case to be the same person (see the Preface). However, in some instances, that practice is unavoidable. At some state and county psychiatric hospitals, for example, treating FMHPs must sometimes testify for (or against) their own patients, or clients, for institutional staffing and budget reasons. In other such examples, a regular roster of FMHPs may be maintained strictly as consultants (i.e., not as treating clinicians), generally for evaluation and testimony on behalf of the state, not the patient or client. While expedient, these practices challenge the concept of the FMHP consultant expert's neutrality, in that the expert is an employee of the retaining agency, with a financial interest in continuing to be employed by that agency, and therefore in the matter in which they are testifying.

practices allow us to maintain a lucrative but ethical practice, as described in the above epigraph.

Table 8.1 gives several aphorisms and caveats relevant to billing and collection procedures for the FMHP consultant from the consultant's and attorney's perspectives. Table 8.2 presents a financial requirements schedule, which has been very helpful to this author in his practice over the years.

TABLE 8.1 Collecting Your Fees

EXPERT	ATTORNEY
▪ *Don't wait* until the case is over: Retainer! Retainer! Retainer!	▪ "Don't worry about your expert fee, Doctor. My client is responsible for it, not me."
	▪ "Doctor, I know my client hasn't paid the balance of your fee. But I have to serve your report/have you testify tomorrow. *Please!*"

TABLE 8.2   Sample Retainer Agreement

RETAINER AGREEMENT / FINANCIAL REQUIREMENTS

Our charges for testimony at trials, depositions, and hearings are

_____ DOLLARS ($_____) per hour.

Our charges are _____ DOLLARS ($_____) per hour
for all other case-related activities, including (but not limited to) record review,
research, interview/evaluation time, and travel time (portal to portal).

Since we anticipate at least 18–20 hours of work on a case, WE REQUIRE A RETAINER OF

_____ DOLLARS ($_____) PRIOR TO COMMENCING WORK.

If less time is expended, we will refund the balance on a pro rata basis.
If more time is experienced, we bill for the difference.

PAYMENT FOR THIS DIFFERENCE (BALANCE DUE) MUST BE RECEIVED
WITHIN SEVEN (7) WORKING DAYS **AFTER RECEIPT** OF THE BILL.

**PLEASE NOTE THAT THE INITIAL RETAINER IS A DEPOSIT ONLY
AND MAY NOT REPRESENT THE ENTIRE FEE.**

If we schedule time for an examination and the examinee does not appear for the
examination or notifies this office of their cancellation fewer than seven (7) working
days before the scheduled examination, then the full charge for the reserved time will
be made.

Concerning depositions (by opposing counsel), and testimony at trial and/or hearing
(by retaining counsel), we require a retainer in advance of anticipated testimony of

_____ DOLLARS ($_____) for the entire day, or

_____ DOLLARS ($_____) for the afternoon
(one half-day), depending on which of these two time periods is reserved.

(It is assumed that two (2) hours travel time will be required.)

This retainer must be received no fewer than **seven** (7) **working days** prior to the
first scheduled date of trial, deposition, or hearing. If the deposition continues,
additional full or half-days must be reserved and paid in the same fashion.

There will be **no refunds** for any time reserved for depositions, hearings, and/or trials
that is not used.

Out-of-pocket expenses (such as travel costs, the costs of psychological test scoring
and interpretation, and so forth), if any, are billed separately as additional charges to
the above and on the same payment schedule.

THE RESPONSIBILITY OF ALL FEES IS ASSUMED BY AND BILLED TO THE LAW
FIRM, **NOT THE CLIENT**: IT IS THE ATTORNEY'S RESPONSIBILITY TO MAKE
WHATEVER ARRANGEMENTS ARE NECESSARY (e.g., ESCROW ACCOUNTS), TO BE
REIMBURSED BY THE CLIENT.

$_____ DUE ON SIGNING:_____ (Date)

Federal Tax ID # _____

Without doubt, the most important aphorism here is "Retainer! Retainer! Retainer!" when obtaining a reasonable retainer in advance of consultation on the case is possible.[3] From both a financial and psychological perspective, retainers are the best option: With retainers, the FMHP consultant no longer has a financial interest in the outcome of the case (until the retainer account runs out) and can maintain their neutrality and objectivity. Also, the FHMP consultant does not have to be concerned about battling counsel about money.[4]

After testimony is complete, and the FMHP consultant/expert has been excused by the court, the expert's last bill to counsel (or the court) has been paid, and no further services are needed, the consultant may consider the case over.

While it may be tempting for the consultant to shred the case file at this point, that practice is inadvisable, since cases have a way of "coming back" in future years. This can occur due to appeals from the underlying case, at which the FMHP consultant may be asked to consult or testify again, to requests from counsel in new cases for case information and materials felt potentially relevant to the new matter; and to requests from treating clinicians for past information and materials about the evaluee felt to be potentially useful for treatment (in which case, the request should be forwarded to the counsel who had retained the FMHP consultant in the first place, since the information and materials were provided for consultation purposes to counsel, and not for clinical purposes to counsel's client). As a practical matter, since FMHP consultants' records and record maintenance (such as federal HIPAA requirements) are carefully articulated by the consultants' professional practice regulatory boards (such as medicine, psychology, counseling, nursing, social work, and so forth), the consultant is well advised to follow those clinical guidelines and requirements for forensic case-related materials.[5] For example, in New Jersey, practitioners' medical records must be maintained for seven years after completion of treatment, a requirement which this author follows for his forensic case consultation records.

---

3 In my experience, this is generally not possible in public sector matters. In last-minute private sector matters, the FMHP's patience may be tried by aggressive counsel who presses for services (such as a report; see Table 8.1) before payment is made, in full or in part. In such situations, counsel will sometimes assure the unpaid expert that if the service is provided before full or partial payment is made, "more cases will be sent your way." My response to that poorly disguised bribe has been "Will those cases also be gratis?"

4 Or counsel's client, which counsel would prefer, but which is not advisable. The FHMP consultant's financial relationship is with counsel, and not with counsel's client.

5 These suggestions are not intended as applicable (e.g., legal) professional advice. Such information is well beyond the nature and scope of this chapter, and the formal training and competence of this author. For further information and details in this area, the reader is referred to applicable professional (legal) advice and consultation, and to applicable professional/legal guidelines, requirements, and documentation.

CHAPTER 9

Wrapping Up

My necessaries are embark'd: farewell!
—William Shakespeare, *Hamlet*

T HE COURT HAS now excused the FMHP expert witness after their testimony is complete, all of the expert's bills and charges have been
paid, and, for all intents and purposes, the case is over for the expert.
What remains?

As a practical matter, after the expert has completed whatever
record-keeping ("If it isn't written down, it didn't happen") is necessary for
the case—for documentation, practice statistics, financial records, and the
like—the case is over, at least for the moment, and the FMHP consultant
may retire the case and archive the related materials.[1] The FMHP consultant
may want to retain materials generated by their evaluation for research, academic (teaching and writing), future consulting, and other such purposes,
while shredding or returning records, materials, and discovery provided by
counsel or the court. In my experience, some FMHP experts/consultants
do, and some do not: It is a matter of personal and professional choice.

A summary of the salient features, suggestions, aphorisms, and caveats
provided in this book follows. These "Pearls, Pitfalls, and Pet Peeves for
Expert Witnesses" (see Table 9.1, below) include, in no particular order,
some of the aphorisms and caveats already presented and discussed in
the book, as well as additional warnings and suggestions, all useful for
conducting an effective and efficient forensic mental health professional
consulting practice.

---

1 But the FMHP consultant should allow for the possibility of appeals, retrials, or retention
of the FHMP consultant for a related case—such as a civil action arising from a resolved
criminal one, as in *The People of the State of California v. O.J. Simpson*—as a reason not to dis-
card files after the minimum required retention period is over. To avoid the accumulation of
excessive amounts of paper and other records, a letter to retaining counsel or the courts several weeks after the conclusion of the case, along the lines of the following, is advisable: *Dear
Counsel: If we do not hear from you within four (4) weeks of our sending you this letter, we will cull
and archive this file. Culling* here refers to the destruction (or return to counsel or the court) of
records initially sent by counsel or the court "to assist you in your evaluation" (see Table 2.3).
Records and materials generated by the FMHP consultant during the course of their evaluation should be kept for as long as professional laws and guidelines require (see Chapter 8).

TABLE 9.1 Pearls, Pitfalls and Pet Peeves for Expert Witnesses

- Cell phones: Beware of poor communication.

- You are the next-to-last step in the food chain, often an afterthought, with difficult last-minute time constraints. Be aware of that and be prepared to deal with the attendant frustration. The situation is *not* going to change!

- Get yourself subpoenaed or court-ordered out of commitments but be sure to resolve payment issues when subpoenaed (you have a "property interest" in your time and your opinion).

- Retainers! Retainers! Retainers!

- Make referrals and cross-referrals to colleagues in other disciplines: Teamwork is important in this work, especially in serious criminal matters (such as death penalty cases).

- Fax: Proof and time of service or non-service (very useful).

- What trumps what: Criminal Trials > Civil Trials > Hearings > Depositions > Court-Ordered Evaluations > Routine Evaluations > Paperwork and Report Writing.

- Articles: Make your own authority. Write about (and publish) things you *do* want to do (e.g., transfer records safely) or *do not* want to do (e.g., testify about blackouts).

- Fee agreements: *In advance*, and *in writing* (including a fee schedule).

- First consultation call–free. Send materials: current CV, financial requirements schedules; provide additional information afterward.

- Testifying: Be pleasant, responsive, engaging, and likeable. Dress carefully, but not lavishly (e.g., wear a conservative "law-suit"). Use the bathroom PRN ("Go early, go often").

- "If there's bad law, argue the facts; if there're bad facts, argue the law; if there's neither, attack the expert." (An old saw.)

- Common sense rules: Testify that way, and do not be afraid to respond to questions that are implied and not directly asked, to make a point.

- Good authority and a definition of medical "standard of care" (malpractice/professional liability context) do not exist. Do not be afraid to assert your own definition and opinions.

- (Overheard from a senior attorney in court): "We lawyers have only one clock: It's the last-minute clock." Advice for the expert witness: Get used to it, because it is not going to change!

- Do not confuse *legal* levels of "burdens of proof" (i.e., "preponderance of the evidence;" "clean and convincing evidence;" and "beyond a reasonable doubt") with the clinical. A scientist offers an opinion with a reasonable degree of probability or certainty, which is then taken into consideration by the trier of fact (judge; jury) in deciding whether the *legal* "burden of proof" is met for the particular case.

- If asked questions during testimony that are not specifically addressed in your evaluation, and if it does not suit your purposes to respond to those questions, *do not* respond to them. Say instead, "I have no opinion about that issue; it is not something that I was asked to address in this evaluation." *You* control responses to questions that implied and not directly asked (see above), *not* counsel.

EPILOGUE

So long, and thanks for all the fish.
—Douglas Adams (1984)[1]

I N CONCLUSION, I hope that this short collection of aphorisms and cave-ats has been helpful, amusing, and informative to its readers as a guide to and overview of the process and pitfalls of conducting a forensic mental health consultation practice.

As I have emphasized before, this book is not intended as an ency-clopedic, scholarly, or detailed "cookbook" of forensic mental health consultation practice. The Selected References in the Preface of this book can serve that purpose, as can many other such works.

But if the reader pays attention to the aphorisms and caveats—and their commentary—presented in this book, then some of the problems and land mines in this potentially difficult practice may be avoided, that the reader may not have to *lasciate ogni speranza, voi ch'entrata* ("abandon all hope, ye who enter here").

Finally, since the success or failure of this book will depend on its use-fulness to its readers, I welcome feedback and suggestions to make future editions as practical and useful as possible.

Please contact me with feedback and suggestions at this email address: dpgreenfieldmdpsychiatry@msn.com.

---

1   Adams, D. (1984). *So long, and thanks for all the fish. (Hitchhiker's Guide to the Galaxy #4).* Pan Books. London, UK. The title of this book is derived from the text of the novel: It is the message left by the dolphins when they departed Planet Earth just before Planet Earth was demolished to make way for a hyperspace bypass.

INDEX

CPSIA information can be obtained
at www.ICGtesting.com
Printed in the USA
LVHW080800261021
701502LV00002B/7